Low Sodium Cooking Guide for Beginners

A Collection of Delicious Low Sodium
Recipes for Your Daily Meals

Jennifer Loyel

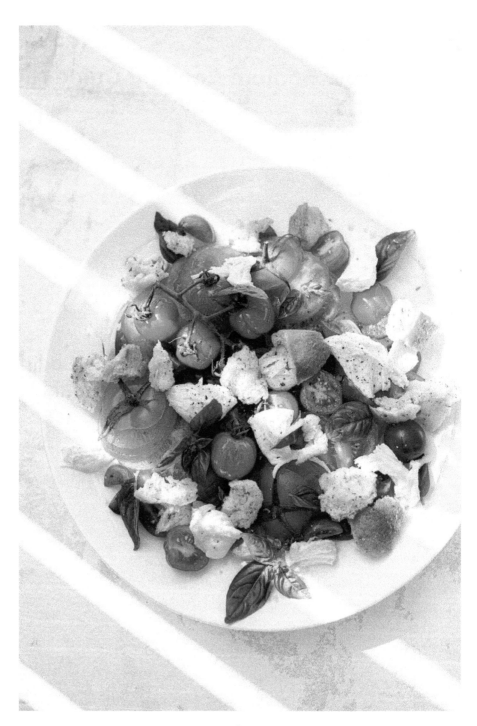

professional advice. The content within this book has been derived from various sources. Please consult a licensed professional before attempting any techniques outlined in this book.

By reading this document, the reader agrees that under no circumstances is the author responsible for any losses, direct or indirect, which are incurred as a result of the use of information contained within this document, including, but not limited to, — errors, omissions, or inaccuracies.

Table of Contents

ICE CREAM SHERBET BUNDT CAKE...................... 9

PUMPKIN PIE FILLING........................... 11

TOFU SMOOTHIES............................... 13

LEMON MERINGUE ANGEL FOOD DESSERT........ 14

PEANUT FUDGE POPS........................... 16

CREAM PUFFS WITH RASPBERRY ICE CREAM..... 18

GRAHAM CRACKERS 20

PEANUT BUTTER S'MORES BARS 22

GRILLED STRAWBERRY SHORTCAKE.................. 24

EASY NO-CRUST APPLE PIE 26

BAKED APPLES WITH WALNUTS 28

BAKED PEARS WITH ROSEMARY 30

CRANBERRY-ORANGE SMOOTHIE..................... 32

APPLE CIDER CUPCAKES 33

MERINGUE COOKIES 35

VIRGIN BELLINI 37

RASPBERRY ICE CREAM 38

APPLE CIDER FROSTING 39

APPLE PEACH CRISP 40

STEAMED RASPBERRY LEMON CUSTARD 42

MOCHA BROWNIES 44

FUNNEL CAKES 47

FRUIT CUP WITH CREAMY DRESSING 49

TOFFEE SQUARES.. 51

LACE COOKIES 53

RED VELVET CUPCAKES....................................... 55

TRIPLE FRUIT MOLD 58

LEMON PEAR CRISP 60

HERBED SUGAR COOKIES 62

DEVIL'S FOOD CAKE.. 64

STRAWBERRY PIE 66

LIME FIZZ 67

HIDDEN SURPRISE CAKES 68

WALNUT CARAMEL APPLE PIZZA 70

PEANUT BUTTER BROWNIES............................... 72

BUTTERSCOTCH PUDDING 74

APPLE CAKE 76

BROWNIES... 78

ANGEL FOOD CAKE... 80

CHOCOLATE CRACKLES 82

CRANBERRY UPSIDE-DOWN CAKE 84

STRAWBERRY BASIL PIE 86

V6.. 87

BLACKBERRY COBBLER 88

COOKIE PIE CRUST 90

STRAWBERRY ICED TEA FIZZ.............................. 92

STRAWBERRY SMOOTHIE 94

TRIPLE BERRY PAVLOVA.................................. 95

PIE CRUST 97

TOMATO JUICE...................................... 98

STRAWBERRY RHUBARB RASPBERRY CRISP...... 99

SNICKERDOODLES 101

BAKED APPLES.. 103

FRUIT SAUCE 105

VENISON AND VEGGIE STOVETOP CASSEROLE 106

PORK TENDERLOIN BRUSCHETTA 109

Ice Cream Sherbet Bundt Cake

Servings: 16

Ingredients:

- 2 quarts ice cream of various flavors
- 1 quart sherbet of various flavors
- 1/2 cup marshmallow crème

Directions:

1. Layer the ice cream, sherbet, and marshmallow crème in the bundt pan, pressing down firmly so there are no air pockets.
2. Cover pan and freeze for at least 8 hours, preferably overnight.
3. An hour before you're ready to serve, remove pan from the freezer. Cover it with hot towels and shake until the ice cream mixture is loosened. Invert onto a serving tray, remove the pan, and immediately refreeze the "cake."
4. Remove from the freezer 10 minutes before serving to make the "cake" easier to slice.

Nutrition Info: (Per Serving):Calories: 215; Total Fat: 8 g; Saturated Fat: 5 g; Cholesterol: 22 mg; Protein: 3

g; Sodium: 72 mg; Potassium: 200 mg; Fiber: 1 g; Carbohydrates: 35 g; Sugar: 28 g

Pumpkin Pie Filling

Servings: 8

Ingredients:

- 1 ¼ cups (281 g) pumpkin, cooked and mashed
- ¾ cup (150 g) sugar
- ¼ teaspoon ground ginger
- 1 teaspoon ground cinnamon
- 1 teaspoon all-purpose flour
- 2 eggs
- 1 cup (235 ml) evaporated milk
- 2 tablespoons (28 ml) water
- ½ teaspoon vanilla extract

Directions:

1. Combine pumpkin, sugar, spices, and flour in a mixing bowl. Add eggs and mix well. Add milk, water, and vanilla. Mix. Pour into pie shell. Bake at 400°F (200°C, gas mark 6) for 45 to 50 minutes or until knife inserted near center comes out clean.

Nutrition Info: (Per Serving): 73 g water; 152 calories (23% from fat, 11% from protein, 66% from carb); 4 g protein; 4 g total fat; 2 g saturated fat; 1 g monounsaturated fat; 0 g polyunsaturated fat; 26 g carb; 1 g fiber; 20 g sugar; 104 mg calcium; 1 mg iron; 56 mg sodium; 197 mg potassium; 196 IU vitamin A; 2 mg vitamin C; 70 mg cholesterol

Tofu Smoothies

Servings: 2

Ingredients:

- 6 ounces (170 g) tofu
- 1 banana
- 1 cup (155 g) cantaloupe, cubed
- ½ cup (120 ml) skim milk
- ½ cup (120 ml) apple juice

Directions:

1. Place all ingredients in blender and process until smooth.

Nutrition Info: (Per Serving): 319 g water; 197 calories (13% from fat, 16% from protein, 72% from carb); 8 g protein; 3 g total fat; 1 g saturated fat; 1 g monounsaturated fat; 1 g polyunsaturated fat; 37 g carb; 3 g fiber; 24 g sugar; 130 mg calcium; 1 mg iron; 60 mg sodium; 845 mg potassium; 3166 IU vitamin A; 40 mg vitamin C; 1 mg cholesterol

Lemon Meringue Angel Food Dessert

Servings: 12

Ingredients:

- 1 Angel Food Cake , cut into cubes
- 11/4 cups heavy whipping cream
- 1/3 cup powdered sugar
- 1 teaspoon vanilla
- 2 cups Lemon Curd
- 1/4 cup finely ground hard lemon candies
- 4 egg whites
- 1 tablespoon lemon juice
- 2/3 cup granulated sugar

Directions:

1. Place cake cubes in a bowl, cover, and set aside.

2. In large bowl, beat whipping cream with powdered sugar and vanilla until stiff peaks form. Fold in lemon curd.

3. Layer the cake cubes and lemon mixture in a 13" × 9" glass baking pan, pressing the cake down slightly so it is all covered with the lemon mixture. Sprinkle with crushed candies.

Cover and refrigerate while you prepare the meringue.

4.   For meringue, combine egg whites, lemon juice, and granulated sugar in the top of a double boiler. Place on a pan of simmering water, making sure the bottom of the double boiler doesn't touch the water below. Stir with a wire whisk until the sugar dissolves.

5.   Beat with a hand mixer until the mixture is stiff and glossy and a thermometer registers 160°F. This should take about 10–15 minutes.

6.   Remove the dessert from the refrigerator and top with the meringue, spreading to cover and sealing the edges.

7.   Preheat oven to broil. Place the dessert 6" from heat source and broil for about 2 minutes, watching carefully, until the meringue is browned on the peaks.

Refrigerate for at least 4 hours before serving.

Nutrition Info: (Per Serving):Calories: 389; Total Fat: 14 g; Saturated Fat: 8 g; Cholesterol: 97 mg; Protein: 4 g; Sodium: 51 mg; Potassium: 129 mg; Fiber: 0 g; Carbohydrates: 62 g; Sugar: 51 g

Peanut Fudge Pops

Servings: 8 Pops

Ingredients:

- 3 tablespoons unsalted butter
- 1/3 cup flour
- 2 cups milk
- 2/3 cup brown sugar
- 3 tablespoons cocoa
- 1/2 cup semisweet chocolate chips
- 1/3 cup unsalted peanut butter
- 1 teaspoon vanilla
- 1/2 cup chopped unsalted peanuts

Directions:

1. In medium saucepan, melt butter over medium heat. Add flour; cook and stir for 1 minute.
2. Add milk, brown sugar, and cocoa; cook, stirring constantly with a wire whisk, until thickened.
3. Add chocolate chips and peanut butter; cook and stir until melted.
4. Remove from heat and add vanilla. Let cool for 1 hour, stirring a few times with the whisk.

16

5. Pour 1/3 cup into each pop mold or 4-ounce paper cup. Add wooden sticks, then sprinkle with peanuts. Freeze until firm.

Nutrition Info: (Per Serving):Calories: 344; Total Fat: 19 g; Saturated Fat: 5 g; Cholesterol: 16 mg; Protein: 8 g; Sodium: 33 mg; Potassium: 283 mg; Fiber: 3 g; Carbohydrates: 39 g; Sugar: 29 g

Cream Puffs With Raspberry Ice Cream

Servings: 6

Ingredients:

- 2/3 cup water
- 1/3 cup unsalted butter
- 2/3 cup flour
- 2 large eggs
- 1 egg white
- 2 teaspoons vanilla
- 6 cups Raspberry Ice Cream
- 1 cup fresh raspberries

Directions:

1. Preheat oven to 400°F. Line baking sheets with parchment paper and set aside.
2. In medium saucepan, combine water and butter and bring to a rolling boil over high heat. Turn heat down to medium, add flour, and beat until a ball forms that cleans the sides of the pan. Remove from heat.
3. Add eggs and the egg white, one at a time, beating well after each addition until mixture is smooth and shiny. Beat in vanilla.

4. Drop batter by 1/4-cup measures onto prepared baking sheets, about 4" apart. Bake for 25–35 minutes or until puffs are golden brown and firm to the touch.
5. Remove puffs from oven and cut a small slit in the top of each one; return to oven for 2 minutes. Let cool on wire racks.
6. When ready to eat, cut puffs in half crosswise. Remove any dough from the inside so you have hollow shells. Fill with ice cream; replace tops, and serve with raspberries.

Nutrition Info: (Per Serving):Calories: 675; Total Fat: 39 g; Saturated Fat: 24 g; Cholesterol: 200 mg; Protein: 11 g; Sodium: 140 mg; Potassium: 480 mg; Fiber: 5 g; Carbohydrates: 70 g; Sugar: 51 g

Graham Crackers

Servings: 36 Graham Crackers

Ingredients:

- 3/4 cup unsalted butter, softened
- 1/2 cup dark brown sugar
- 1/4 cup light brown sugar
- 1/3 cup honey
- 2 teaspoons vanilla
- 1/2 cup milk
- 1/4 cup water
- 3 cups whole-wheat pastry flour
- 11/2 cups all-purpose flour
- 1 teaspoon baking powder
- 1/4 teaspoon baking soda
- 1/2 teaspoon cinnamon
- 1/8 teaspoon nutmeg

Directions:

1. In large bowl, combine butter and brown sugars; beat until fluffy. Add honey, beating until fluffy. Beat in vanilla, milk, and water.

2. Sift together pastry flour, all-purpose flour, baking powder, baking soda, cinnamon, and nutmeg and add to creamed mixture.

3. Cover dough and refrigerate overnight.

4. When you're ready to bake, preheat oven to 350°F. Roll the dough into 1" balls, using floured hands, and place 4" apart on baking sheet. Press down with a glass or a spatula to make thin rounds. Prick each round with a fork.

5. Bake for 12–15 minutes or until the crackers are set and no imprint remains when lightly touched with your finger. Let cool for 5 minutes on baking sheets, then cool completely on wire racks.

Nutrition Info: (Per Serving):Calories: 116; Total Fat: 4 g; Saturated Fat: 2 g; Cholesterol: 10 mg; Protein: 2 g; Sodium: 22 mg; Potassium: 60 mg; Fiber: 1 g; Carbohydrates: 18 g; Sugar: 7 g

Peanut Butter S'mores Bars

Servings: 36 Bar Cookies

Ingredients:

- 1/2 cup unsalted butter, melted
- 1 cup unsalted peanut butter, divided
- 2 cups Graham Crackers crumbs
- 1/2 cup chopped unsalted peanuts
- 4 cups mini marshmallows
- 1 (12-ounce) package semisweet chocolate chips

Directions:

1. Preheat oven to 350°F. Spray a 13" × 9" pan with nonstick baking spray containing flour.
2. In large bowl, combine unsalted butter, 1/2 cup peanut butter, graham cracker crumbs, and unsalted peanuts and mix until combined. Press into bottom of baking pan.
3. Bake for 12–14 minutes or until crust is set. Remove from oven and sprinkle with marshmallows; turn oven to broil.
4. Put the pan under the broiler; watching carefully, broil until the marshmallows puff and start to turn brown, turning pan

occasionally. Remove from oven and place on wire rack.

5.   In small bowl, combine chocolate chips and remaining 1/2 cup peanut butter; microwave on high for 2 minutes. Remove from microwave and stir. Continue microwaving for 30-second intervals, stirring after each, until mixture is smooth. Pour over marshmallows. Let stand until set, then cut into bars.

Nutrition Info: (Per Serving):Calories: 190; Total Fat: 11 g; Saturated Fat: 3 g; Cholesterol: 11 mg; Protein: 4 g; Sodium: 16 mg; Potassium: 87 mg; Fiber: 1 g; Carbohydrates: 20 g; Sugar: 12 g

Grilled Strawberry Shortcake

Servings: 6

Ingredients:

- 3/4 cup heavy whipping cream
- 1/4 cup powdered sugar
- 1/4 cup Lemon Curd
- 2 cups strawberries
- 6 slices Angel Food Cake

Directions:

1. In medium bowl, combine whipping cream with powdered sugar; beat until soft peaks form. Fold in the lemon curd, cover, and refrigerate.

2. Prepare and preheat grill. Remove the stems and leaves from the strawberries and wash gently; pat dry. Place strawberries in a grill basket.

3. Grill the berries for a minute or two until they are warm. Remove from grill basket and let cool. Crush 1/2 cup of the strawberries in a small bowl. Slice remaining strawberries in about 1/4" slices.

4.   Grill the angel food cake for a minute or two on each side until grill marks form. Place cake slices on serving plates.

5.   Drizzle with the crushed strawberries and top with sliced strawberries. Top with the whipped-cream mixture and serve immediately.

Nutrition Info: (Per Serving):Calories: 309; Total Fat: 12 g; Saturated Fat: 7 g; Cholesterol: 56 mg; Protein: 2 g; Sodium: 21 mg; Potassium: 180 mg; Fiber: 1 g; Carbohydrates: 48 g; Sugar: 36 g

Easy No-crust Apple Pie

Servings: 8

Ingredients:

- 4 apples, peeled
- 1 tablespoon (7 g) ground cinnamon
- 1 tablespoon (13 g) sugar
- 1 egg
- ¾ cup (165 g) unsalted butter, melted
- ½ cup (100 g) sugar
- ½ teaspoon sodium-free baking powder
- 1 cup (110 g) all-purpose flour

Directions:

1. Slice the apples into a bowl. Add cinnamon and 1 tablespoon (13 g) sugar and mix well. Dump into a greased 10-inch (25-cm) glass pie plate. In the same bowl beat the egg, add melted butter, ½ cup

2. (100 g) sugar, baking powder, and flour. Pour over apples (it'll be thick, so I actually put little spoonfuls all over to make sure it all gets covered). Bake at 350°F (180°C, gas mark 4) for 40 to 45 minutes until golden

brown and a toothpick inserted comes out clean.

Nutrition Info: (Per Serving): 67 g water; 308 calories (52% from fat, 4% from protein, 44% from carb); 3 g protein; 18 g total fat; 11 g saturated fat; 5 g monounsaturated fat; 1 g polyunsaturated fat; 35 g carb; 2 g fiber; 21 g sugar; 39 mg calcium; 1 mg iron; 13 mg sodium; 125 mg potassium; 594 IU vitamin A; 3 mg vitamin C; 76 mg cholesterol

Baked Apples With Walnuts

Servings: 6

Ingredients:

- 6 apples
- 6 tablespoons (90 g) brown sugar
- ½ cup (75 g) unsalted walnuts, chopped
- ½ teaspoon ground cinnamon
- ½ teaspoon ground nutmeg
- 6 teaspoons (30 g) unsalted butter
- ⅔ cup (157 ml) apple cider or juice

Directions:

1. Core apples carefully so that the cavity is a decent size, but do not cut all the way through the bottom of the apple. Put 1 tablespoon (15 g) brown sugar in each apple, then divide walnuts evenly between the apple cavities. Sprinkle cinnamon and nutmeg over the walnuts, and add a teaspoon of butter to each cavity. Set the apples in an ovenproof baking dish and pour hot cider or juice around the apples. Bake in a preheated 375°F (190°C, gas mark 5) oven for 50 to 60 minutes, or until tender, basting occasionally.

Nutrition Info: (Per Serving): 137 g water; 226 calories (38% from fat, 5% from protein, 57% from carb); 3 g protein; 10 g total fat; 3 g saturated fat; 3 g monounsaturated fat; 4 g polyunsaturated fat; 34 g carb; 3 g fiber; 29 g sugar; 30 mg calcium; 1 mg iron; 7 mg sodium; 253 mg potassium; 172 IU vitamin A; 6 mg vitamin C; 10 mg cholesterol

Baked Pears With Rosemary

Servings: 4

Ingredients:

- 2 large pears, peeled, cored, and cut in half
- 2 tablespoons unsalted butter
- 2 tablespoons brown sugar
- 1 tablespoon granulated sugar
- 2 tablespoons honey
- 1 tablespoon lemon juice
- 1 teaspoon minced fresh rosemary leaves

Directions:

1. Preheat oven to 400°F. Place the pears, cut side up, in a 2-quart baking dish and set aside.

2. In small saucepan, combine butter, brown sugar, granulated sugar, honey, lemon juice, and rosemary. Cook over low heat, stirring frequently, until sugar melts.

3. Drizzle this mixture over the pears. Bake for 20–30 minutes until pears are tender when pierced with a fork. Serve with rosemary

leaves and whipped cream or ice cream, if desired.

Nutrition Info: (Per Serving):Calories: 181; Total Fat: 5 g; Saturated Fat: 3 g; Cholesterol: 15 mg; Protein: 0 g; Sodium: 3 mg; Potassium: 156 mg; Fiber: 3 g; Carbohydrates: 34 g; Sugar: 27 g

Cranberry-orange Smoothie

Servings: 2

Ingredients:

- ½ cup (125 g) cranberry sauce
- ½ cup (120 ml) orange juice
- 1 cup (230 g) plain low-fat yogurt
- 1 banana
- ½ cup (120 ml) skim milk

Directions:

1. Combine all ingredients in blender and process until smooth.

Nutrition Info: (Per Serving): 312 g water; 301 calories (7% from fat, 13% from protein, 79% from carb); 10 g protein; 3 g total fat; 1 g saturated fat; 1 g monounsaturated fat; 0 g polyunsaturated fat; 62 g carb; 3 g fiber; 44 g sugar; 325 mg calcium; 1 mg iron; 143 mg sodium; 803 mg potassium; 313 IU vitamin A; 30 mg vitamin C; 9 mg cholesterol

Apple Cider Cupcakes

Servings: 18

Ingredients:

- 3 cups (705 ml) apple cider
- ¼ cup (165 g) unsalted butter
- 1 ¾ cups (350 g) sugar
- 2 eggs
- 2 cups (220 g) all-purpose flour
- ⅛ teaspoon ground cloves
- 1 teaspoon ground cinnamon
- 1 teaspoon sodium-free baking soda

Directions:

1. In a large saucepan, boil the cider until it is reduced to about 1 ½ cups (355 ml) and let it cool. In a large bowl, beat together the butter and the sugar with an electric mixer until the mixture is fluffy. Beat in the eggs. Into the bowl sift together the flour, the cloves, the cinnamon, and the baking soda; stir in the reduced cider and Combine the mixture well. Divide the batter among 18 paper-lined muffin tins and bake in the middle of a preheated

375°F (190°C, gas mark 5) oven for 25 minutes, or until a tester comes out clean.

Nutrition Info: (Per Serving): 45 g water; 224 calories (34% from fat, 4% from protein, 62% from carb); 2 g protein; 9 g total fat; 5 g saturated fat; 2 g monounsaturated fat; 0 g polyunsaturated fat; 35 g carb; 0 g fiber; 24 g sugar; 13 mg calcium; 1 mg iron; 12 mg sodium; 76 mg potassium; 269 IU vitamin A; 0 mg vitamin C; 48 mg cholesterol

Meringue Cookies

Servings: 48 Cookies

Ingredients:

- 2/3 cup sugar
- 2 egg whites
- 1/8 teaspoon cream of tartar
- 1/16 teaspoon lemon juice
- 1/2 teaspoon vanilla

Directions:

1. Preheat oven to 300°F. Line a cookie sheet with parchment paper and set aside. Place the sugar in a blender or food processor and blend or process until it is finely ground.

2. In medium bowl, combine egg whites, cream of tartar, and lemon juice, and beat with a mixer until soft peaks form.

3. Gradually add the sugar, beating with mixer on high until the mixture is stiff and glossy. The sugar should be almost dissolved when you feel a bit of the meringue between your fingers. Beat in vanilla.

4. Drop by heaping teaspoons onto prepared cookie sheet. Bake for 25–35 minutes or until

the meringues are firm to the touch. Turn off oven, open door, and cool for 30 minutes. Then transfer the paper with the cookies to a wire rack and cool completely. Store in an airtight container at room temperature.

Nutrition Info: (Per Serving):Calories: 11; Total Fat: 0 g; Saturated Fat: 0 g; Cholesterol: 0 mg; Protein: 0 g; Sodium: 2 mg; Potassium: 3 mg; Fiber: 0 g; Carbohydrates: 2 g; Sugar: 2 g

Virgin Bellini

Servings: 4

Ingredients:

- 2 large peaches, peeled, pitted, and cubed
- 1 tablespoon honey
- Optional: Drop of natural almond extract or flavoring or food-grade peppermint oil
- Ice cubes
- Seltzer water
- Optional: Mint sprigs

Directions:

1. In a blender or food processor, combine the peaches, honey, and almond extract or flavoring, if using; process until puréed.
2. Divide among 4 champagne flutes or tall glasses filled with ice cubes. Add enough seltzer water to fill the glasses, and stir. Garnish the glasses with fresh mint, if desired. Serve immediately.

Nutrition Info: (Per Serving):Calories: 50; Total Fat: 0 g; Saturated Fat: 0 g; Cholesterol: 0 mg; Protein: 0 g; Sodium: 0 mg; Potassium: 168 mg; Fiber: 1 g; Carbohydrates: 12 g; Sugar: 11 g

Raspberry Ice Cream

Servings: 12

Ingredients:

- 1 (14-ounce) can sweetened condensed milk
- 11/2 cups heavy whipping cream
- 2 tablespoons lemon juice
- 1 teaspoon vanilla
- 11/2 cups frozen raspberries, thawed
- 1 cup fresh raspberries

Directions:

1. In large bowl, combine sweetened condensed milk, cream, lemon juice, and vanilla. Beat with a mixer until soft peaks form.
2. Fold in the frozen raspberries to marble, then the fresh raspberries. Pour into a freezer container and freeze until firm, about 4–6 hours.

Nutrition Info: (Per Serving):Calories: 248; Total Fat: 14 g; Saturated Fat: 8 g; Cholesterol: 52 mg; Protein: 3 g; Sodium: 53 mg; Potassium: 200 mg; Fiber: 2 g; Carbohydrates: 28 g; Sugar: 25 g

Apple Cider Frosting

Servings: 18

Ingredients:

- ¼ cup (55 g) unsalted butter, softened
- 2 cups (200 g) confectioners' sugar
- 3 tablespoons (45 ml) apple cider

Directions:

1. Beat together butter, sugar, and cider until smooth. Add more cider if necessary to make frosting of spreading consistency.

Nutrition Info: (Per Serving): 3 g water; 76 calories (30% from fat, 0% from protein, 70% from carb); 0 g protein; 3 g total fat; 2 g saturated fat; 1 g monounsaturated fat; 0 g polyunsaturated fat; 14 g carb; 0 g fiber; 13 g sugar; 1 mg calcium; 0 mg iron; 1 mg sodium; 4 mg potassium; 79 IU vitamin A; 0 mg vitamin C; 7 mg cholesterol

Apple Peach Crisp

Servings: 8

Ingredients:

- 3 cups Granny Smith apple slices, peeled, cored, and sliced 1/4" thick
- 2 cups peach slices, peeled, sliced 1/2" thick
- 2 tablespoons lemon juice
- 1 cup granulated sugar, divided
- 2 tablespoons cornstarch
- 1/2 teaspoon cinnamon
- 1/8 teaspoon nutmeg
- 2 cups flour
- 2 cups quick-cooking oats
- 1 cup brown sugar
- 1 cup unsalted butter, melted

Directions:

1. Preheat oven to 350°F. Combine apples and peaches in a 13" × 9" glass baking dish. Sprinkle with lemon juice. In a small bowl, combine 1/2 cup granulated sugar, cornstarch, cinnamon, and nutmeg and sprinkle over fruit; toss to coat.

2.   In large bowl, combine flour, oats, brown sugar, and remaining 1/2 cup granulated sugar and mix well. Add melted butter and mix until crumbly. Sprinkle over fruit in the baking dish.

3.   Bake for 45–55 minutes or until fruit is tender. Remove from oven and let cool for 45 minutes before serving.

Nutrition Info: (Per Serving):Calories: 634; Total Fat: 24 g; Saturated Fat: 14 g; Cholesterol: 60 mg; Protein: 6 g; Sodium: 12 mg; Potassium: 263 mg; Fiber: 3 g; Carbohydrates: 100 g; Sugar: 59 g

Steamed Raspberry Lemon Custard

Servings: 4

Ingredients:

- 2 large eggs
- 1/4 teaspoon cream of tartar
- 1 lemon, zested and juiced
- 1/4 teaspoon pure lemon extract
- 3 tablespoons unbleached all-purpose flour
- 1/4 cup granulated sugar
- 40 fresh raspberries
- Optional: 12 additional fresh raspberries
- Optional: Fresh mint leaves
- Optional: 2–4 teaspoons powdered sugar

Directions:

1. Separate the egg yolks and whites. Add the egg whites to a large bowl and set aside the yolks. Use an electric mixer or wire whisk to beat the egg whites until frothy. Add the cream of tartar; continue to whip or whisk until soft peaks form.

2. In a small bowl, mix together the lemon zest, lemon juice, lemon extract, flour, sugar, and

42

egg yolks; gently fold into the whites with a spatula.

3. Treat 4 (6-ounce) ramekins with nonstick spray. Place 10 raspberries in the bottom of each. Spoon the batter into the ramekins and set them in a steamer with a lid; cover and steam for 15–20 minutes.

4. To remove the custards from the ramekins, run a thin knife around edges; turn upside down onto plates. Garnish with raspberries, mint, and a dusting of powdered sugar, if desired.

Nutrition Info: (Per Serving):Calories: 137; Total Fat: 3 g; Saturated Fat: 0 g; Cholesterol: 105 mg; Protein: 4 g; Sodium: 35 mg; Potassium: 163 mg; Fiber: 4 g; Carbohydrates: 25 g; Sugar: 15 g

Mocha Brownies

Servings: 36 Brownies

Ingredients:

- 1 1/4 cups unsalted butter, divided
- 1/4 cup safflower or peanut oil
- 1 3/4 cups brown sugar, divided
- 1 cup granulated sugar
- 2/3 cup cocoa powder
- 1/2 cup milk chocolate chips
- 4 large eggs
- 3/4 cup flour
- 1 tablespoon espresso powder
- 2 teaspoons vanilla, divided
- 1/2 cup crushed chocolate-covered coffee beans
- 3 tablespoons milk
- 2 cups sifted powdered sugar

Directions:

1. Preheat oven to 325°F. Spray a 13" × 9" baking pan with nonstick baking spray containing flour and set aside.
2. In large saucepan, melt 3/4 cup butter with oil over medium heat. Add 1 cup brown sugar

and granulated sugar and cook, stirring, for 2
minutes.

3.   Add cocoa powder and chocolate chips and
stir for 2 minutes or until chips are melted.
Remove from heat.

4.   Beat in eggs, one at a time, beating well
after each addition. Add flour and espresso
powder and mix well, then stir in 1 teaspoon
vanilla and coffee beans.

5.   Pour into prepared pan. Bake for 22–27
minutes or until brownies are just set and
have a shiny crust. Remove from oven and
cool on wire rack.

6.   For frosting, melt remaining 1/2 cup butter in
small saucepan over medium heat. Add
remaining 3/4 cup brown sugar and stir until
mixture just comes to a boil.

7.   Remove from heat and add milk; stir with
wire whisk until smooth. Beat in powdered
sugar and remaining 1 teaspoon vanilla until
smooth. Pour over brownies and let stand until
set.

Nutrition Info: (Per Serving):Calories: 194; Total Fat:
10 g; Saturated Fat: 5 g; Cholesterol: 41 mg; Protein:

1 g; Sodium: 13 mg; Potassium: 60 mg; Fiber: 0 g; Carbohydrates: 25 g; Sugar: 21 g

Funnel Cakes

Servings: 4

Ingredients:

- 1 egg
- ⅔ cup (157 ml) skim milk
- 1 ¼ cups (145 g) all-purpose flour
- 2 tablespoons (26 g) sugar
- 1 teaspoon sodium-free baking powder
- ¼ cup (25 g) confectioners' sugar

Directions:

1. Beat egg with milk. Blend flour, sugar, and baking powder and gradually add egg mixture, beating until smooth. Heat at least 1 inch (2.5 cm) of oil in skillet or deep fryer to 375°F (190°C, gas mark 5). Place thumb over bottom opening of funnel. Pour batter in. Remove thumb and drop into hot oil using a circular motion to form spirals about 4 inches (10 cm) in diameter for each cake. Remove when golden brown. While cake is still warm, sprinkle with confectioners' sugar. Serve warm.

Nutrition Info: (Per Serving): 52 g water; 235 calories (7% from fat, 13% from protein, 80% from carb); 7 g protein; 2 g total fat; 1 g saturated fat; 1 g monounsaturated fat; 0 g polyunsaturated fat; 47 g carb; 1 g fiber; 14 g sugar; 126 mg calcium; 2 mg iron; 46 mg sodium; 262 mg potassium; 154 IU vitamin A; 0 mg vitamin C; 62 mg cholesterol

Fruit Cup With Creamy Dressing

Servings: 1

Ingredients:

- 1/8 cup peeled and grated carrots
- 1 tablespoon raisins
- 1/4 cup cubed or sliced apple
- 6 seedless red or green grapes
- 4 ounces plain nonfat yogurt
- 1 tablespoon unsweetened, no-salt-added applesauce
- 1 teaspoon lemon juice
- 1/4 teaspoon honey
- 1/8 teaspoon Pumpkin Pie Spice
- 1/8 teaspoon finely grated fresh lemon zest

Directions:

1. Arrange the carrots and fruit in a dessert cup.
2. In a medium bowl, mix the yogurt, applesauce, lemon juice, honey, and pumpkin pie spice together and drizzle over the fruit.
3. Sprinkle lemon zest over the top.

Nutrition Info: (Per Serving):Calories: 158; Total Fat: 0 g; Saturated Fat: 0 g; Cholesterol: 2 mg; Protein: 4 g; Sodium: 99 mg; Potassium: 541 mg; Fiber: 1 g; Carbohydrates: 33 g; Sugar: 28 g

Toffee Squares

Servings: 32 Bar Cookies

Ingredients:

- 3/4 cup unsalted butter, softened
- 1/3 cup brown sugar
- 1/4 cup granulated sugar
- 2 tablespoons powdered sugar
- 11/2 teaspoons vanilla
- 1/4 cup toffee bits, finely crushed
- 11/2 cups flour
- 1 (11.5-ounce) package milk chocolate chips
- 1/2 cup toffee bits
- 1/2 cup chopped toasted pecans

Directions:

1. Preheat oven to 350°F. Spray a 9" × 13" pan with nonstick baking spray containing flour and set aside.
2. In large bowl, combine butter, brown sugar, granulated sugar, powdered sugar, and vanilla and beat until smooth. Stir in finely crushed toffee bits.

3.   Add flour and mix until a dough forms. Press into prepared pan.

4.   Bake for 20–25 minutes or until bars are set and light golden brown. Immediately sprinkle with chocolate chips; cover pan with foil. Let stand 5 minutes, then spread the melted chips over the bars with a knife. Sprinkle with 1/2 cup toffee bits and toasted pecans; let cool completely.

Nutrition Info: (Per Serving):Calories: 164; Total Fat: 10 g; Saturated Fat: 3 g; Cholesterol: 14 mg; Protein: 1 g; Sodium: 18 mg; Potassium: 26 mg; Fiber: 1 g; Carbohydrates: 19 g; Sugar: 12 g

Lace Cookies

Servings: 48 Cookies

Ingredients:

- 1/2 cup unsalted butter
- 3/4 cup brown sugar
- 1/4 cup granulated sugar
- 1 cup rolled oats
- 1/4 cup flour
- 1 tablespoon honey
- 1 tablespoon heavy cream
- 1 teaspoon vanilla

Directions:

1. Preheat oven to 375°F. In large saucepan, melt butter over medium heat. Add brown sugar and granulated sugar and stir until smooth. Stir in rolled oats, flour, honey, heavy cream, and vanilla, beating well.

2. Line cookie sheets with silicone baking mats or parchment paper. Drop the batter onto the lined sheets with a teaspoon, leaving about 3" between each cookie, because they spread while they bake.

3. Bake for 6–7 minutes until golden brown. Remove from oven and set aside for about a minute, then carefully remove to a wire rack to cool. You can drape them over a rolling pin or around a form at this point.

Nutrition Info: (Per Serving):Calories: 45; Total Fat: 2 g; Saturated Fat: 1 g; Cholesterol: 5 mg; Protein: 0 g; Sodium: 1 mg; Potassium: 12 mg; Fiber: 0 g; Carbohydrates: 6 g; Sugar: 4 g

Red Velvet Cupcakes

Servings: 12 Cupcakes

Ingredients:

- 1 large beet
- 1 tablespoon safflower or peanut oil
- 2/3 cup milk
- 2 tablespoons lemon juice
- 13/4 cups all-purpose flour
- 1/4 cup cornstarch
- 2 tablespoons cocoa powder
- 1/8 teaspoon salt
- 1/2 teaspoon baking powder
- 1/4 teaspoon baking soda
- 3/4 cup granulated sugar
- 1/3 cup brown sugar
- 3 large eggs
- 1/2 cup unsalted butter, melted
- 2 teaspoons vanilla, divided
- 4 ounces cream cheese, softened
- 2 tablespoons unsalted butter, softened
- 2 cups powdered sugar

Directions:

1. Preheat oven to 375°F. Line a 12-cup muffin tin with paper liners.

2. Place the beet on a cookie sheet and drizzle with oil. Roast for about 1 hour or until the beet is tender. Remove from oven and let cool completely; peel and chop (use gloves or your hands will be dyed red).

3. Purée beet in a food processor or blender. In small bowl, combine milk and lemon juice; mix and set aside.

4. In a medium bowl, combine flour, cornstarch, cocoa, salt, baking powder, and baking soda, and mix well with a wire whisk.

5. In a large bowl, beat granulated sugar, brown sugar, and eggs until light. Add milk mixture, 1/2 cup melted butter, puréed beets, and 1 1/2 teaspoons vanilla and beat well. Beat in flour mixture just until smooth.

6. Spoon batter into prepared muffin cups. Bake for 25–30 minutes or until cupcakes spring back when lightly touched. Let cool completely on racks.

7. In medium bowl, combine cream cheese, 2
    tablespoons softened butter, powdered sugar,
    and remaining 1/2 teaspoon vanilla and beat
    well. Frost cooled cupcakes.

Nutrition Info: (Per Serving):Calories: 384; Total Fat: 15 g; Saturated Fat: 8 g; Cholesterol: 89 mg; Protein: 4 g; Sodium: 127 mg; Potassium: 121 mg; Fiber: 1 g; Carbohydrates: 57 g; Sugar: 39 g

Triple Fruit Mold

Servings: 6

Ingredients:

- 2 envelopes unflavored gelatin
- 1/2 cup frozen, unsweetened apple juice concentrate
- 3 cups unsweetened sparkling water
- 1 cup sliced strawberries
- 1 cup blueberries
- 2 large bananas, peeled and sliced

Directions:

1. Mix together the gelatin and apple juice in a small saucepan; let stand for 1 minute. Stir the gelatin over low heat until completely dissolved, about 3 minutes. Let cool slightly.

2. Stir in the sparkling water. Refrigerate until the mixture begins to gel or is the consistency of unbeaten egg whites when stirred, about 15 minutes.

3. Fold the fruit into the partially thickened gelatin mixture. Pour into a 6-cup mold. Refrigerate for 4 hours or until set.

Nutrition Info: (Per Serving):Calories: 126; Total Fat: 0 g; Saturated Fat: 0 g; Cholesterol: 0 mg; Protein: 8 g; Sodium: 24 mg; Potassium: 313 mg; Fiber: 2 g; Carbohydrates: 24 g; Sugar: 16 g

Lemon Pear Crisp

Servings: 8

Ingredients:

- 6 large ripe pears, peeled, cored, and sliced
- 2 tablespoons honey
- 1/4 cup sugar
- 1 cup plus 2 tablespoons flour, divided
- 2 tablespoons lemon juice
- 1 teaspoon grated lemon zest
- 2 teaspoons minced fresh thyme leaves
- 11/2 cups rolled oats
- 1 cup brown sugar
- 3/4 cup unsalted butter, melted
- 1 cup chopped walnuts

Directions:

1. Preheat oven to 350°F. Spray a 13" × 9" baking dish with nonstick baking spray containing flour.
2. Place pears in the baking dish. Top with honey, sugar, 2 tablespoons flour, lemon juice, lemon zest, and thyme and toss gently to coat.

60

3. In medium bowl, combine remaining 1 cup flour, rolled oats, and brown sugar and mix well. Add melted butter and stir until crumbly. Add walnuts. Sprinkle over pears in baking pan.

4. Bake for 50–55 minutes or until pears are tender and bubbling around the edges and the topping is golden brown. Cool 30 minutes, then serve.

Nutrition Info: (Per Serving):Calories: 516; Total Fat: 20 g; Saturated Fat: 11 g; Cholesterol: 45 mg; Protein: 5 g; Sodium: 12 mg; Potassium: 296 mg; Fiber: 6 g; Carbohydrates: 82 g; Sugar: 50 g

Herbed Sugar Cookies

Servings: 48 Cookies

Ingredients:

- 1 cup unsalted butter, softened
- 3/4 cup Herbed Sugar
- 1/3 cup powdered sugar
- 1 large egg
- 2 egg whites
- 1/4 cup light cream
- 1/4 teaspoon vanilla
- 22/3 cups flour
- 1/2 teaspoon baking powder
- 1/4 teaspoon baking soda

Directions:

1. Preheat oven to 350°F.
2. In large bowl, combine butter with herbed sugar and powdered sugar; beat well until fluffy.
3. Add egg and beat well, then beat in egg whites. Beat in light cream and vanilla.
4. Add flour, baking powder, and baking soda and mix just until a dough forms. Cover dough and chill for at least 4 hours.

5.   Roll out the dough onto floured work surface to 1/4" thick and cut with cookie cutters. You can also roll the dough into 1" balls; place on ungreased cookie sheets and flatten with a glass or a spatula.

6.   Bake for 8–10 minutes or until the cookies are set and very light gold on the bottom. Let cool on cookie sheets for 2 minutes, then remove to wire rack to cool completely. Frost when cool, if desired.

Nutrition Info: (Per Serving):Calories: 82; Total Fat: 4 g; Saturated Fat: 2 g; Cholesterol: 16 mg; Protein: 1 g; Sodium: 15 mg; Potassium: 14 mg; Fiber: 0 g; Carbohydrates: 9 g; Sugar: 4 g

Devil's Food Cake

Servings: 24

Ingredients:

- 2 cups (220 g) all-purpose flour
- 1 ¾ cups (350 g) sugar
- ½ cup (55 g) unsweetened cocoa powder
- 1 tablespoon (14 g) sodium-free baking soda
- ⅔ cup (147 g) applesauce
- ⅓ cup (80 ml) buttermilk
- 2 tablespoons (30 ml) vegetable oil
- 1 cup (235 ml) coffee

Directions:

1. Preheat oven to 350°F (180°C, gas mark 4). Spray a 9 × 13-inch (23 × 33-cm) pan with nonstick vegetable oil spray and then dust with flour, shaking out the excess. In a large bowl, mix together flour, sugar, cocoa, and baking soda. Stir in the applesauce, buttermilk, and oil. Heat coffee to boiling. Stir into batter. Mixture will be thin. Pour into pan. Bake 35 to 40 minutes, until a toothpick inserted in the center comes out clean.

Nutrition Info: (Per Serving): 20 g water; 116 calories (11% from fat, 5% from protein, 83% from carb); 2 g protein; 2 g total fat; 0 g saturated fat; 0 g monounsaturated fat; 1 g polyunsaturated fat; 25 g carb; 1 g fiber; 15 g sugar; 8 mg calcium; 1 mg iron; 6 mg sodium; 55 mg potassium; 2 IU vitamin A; 0 mg vitamin C; 0 mg cholesterol

Strawberry Pie

Servings: 8

Ingredients:

- 3 cups (510 g) strawberries, sliced
- 1 Pie Crust
- 1 cup (235 ml) water
- 2 tablespoons (16 g) cornstarch
- ½ cup (100 g) sugar
- 1 small box (0.3 ounces) strawberry sugar-free Jell-O or other gelatin dessert powder

Directions:

1. Put sliced berries in pie crust. Combine water, cornstarch, and sugar. Heat until sugar is melted and mixture is clear. Add gelatin and pour over berries. Chill until set.

Nutrition Info: (Per Serving): 86 g water; 188 calories (36% from fat, 4% from protein, 61% from carb); 2 g protein; 8 g total fat; 2 g saturated fat; 3 g monounsaturated fat; 2 g polyunsaturated fat; 29 g carb; 2 g fiber; 15 g sugar; 12 mg calcium; 1 mg iron; 118 mg sodium; 102 mg potassium; 7 IU vitamin A; 34 mg vitamin C; 0 mg cholesterol

Lime Fizz

Servings: 1

Ingredients:

- 2 tablespoons (28 ml) lime juice
- 2 teaspoons (8 g) sugar
- ¼ cup (60 ml) water
- 1 cup (235 ml) seltzer water

Directions:

1. Combine juice, sugar, and water in a tall glass. Stir until dissolved. Add ice. Fill glass with seltzer.

Nutrition Info: (Per Serving): 324 g water; 41 calories (1% from fat, 1% from protein, 98% from carb); 0 g protein; 0 g total fat; 0 g saturated fat; 0 g monounsaturated fat; 0 g polyunsaturated fat; 11 g carb; 0 g fiber; 9 g sugar; 37 mg calcium; 0 mg iron; 4 mg sodium; 34 mg potassium; 15 IU vitamin A; 9 mg vitamin C; 0 mg cholesterol

Hidden Surprise Cakes

Servings: 12

Ingredients:

- 1 cup unbleached all-purpose flour
- 1/8 teaspoon salt
- 1 teaspoon baking powder
- 3 large eggs
- 3/4 cup vanilla sugar
- 1 tablespoon lemon juice
- Optional: 1/2 teaspoon grated lemon zest
- 6 tablespoons hot skim milk
- 1 (1.2-ounce) package dark chocolate peppermint cups
- 1 tablespoon cocoa powder

Directions:

1. Preheat oven to 350°F. Treat a 12-cup muffin pan with nonstick spray or line with foil liners.

2. In a small bowl, mix together the flour, salt, and baking powder. Add the eggs to the bowl of a food processor or a mixing bowl; pulse or beat until fluffy and lemon colored. Add the vanilla sugar, lemon juice, and the optional

lemon zest, if using; pulse or beat to mix. Add the flour mixture; process or mix just enough to blend. Add the hot milk and process or mix until blended.

3. Spoon the batter halfway up the muffin sections in the prepared muffin pan. Cut each peppermint cup into 4 equal pieces. Add 1 piece to each muffin cup. Spoon the remaining batter over the top of the candy.

4. Bake for 15 minutes or until the cakes are light golden brown and firm to touch. Dust the tops of the cakes with cocoa powder. Move to a rack to cool.

Nutrition Info: (Per Serving):Calories: 120; Total Fat: 1 g; Saturated Fat: 0 g; Cholesterol: 53 mg; Protein: 3 g; Sodium: 75 mg; Potassium: 50 mg; Fiber: 0 g; Carbohydrates: 23 g; Sugar: 14 g

Walnut Caramel Apple Pizza

Servings: 8

Ingredients:

- 2 recipes unbaked Cookie Pie Crust
- 4 large apples, peeled and sliced
- 2 tablespoons lemon juice
- 1/4 cup granulated sugar
- 1 teaspoon cinnamon
- 1/8 teaspoon nutmeg or cardamom
- 3/4 cup brown sugar
- 1/2 cup corn syrup
- 3 tablespoons unsalted butter
- 1/4 cup heavy cream
- 1 teaspoon vanilla
- 20 caramels, unwrapped and quartered

Directions:

1. Preheat oven to 375°F. Make the cookie pie crust and press into a metal 13" × 9" baking pan. Bake for 5 minutes or until just set.
2. In large bowl, toss apples with lemon juice, granulated sugar, cinnamon, and nutmeg; set aside.

3. In heavy saucepan, combine brown sugar, corn syrup, and butter and bring to a boil over medium heat. Cook, stirring constantly with a wire whisk, for about 5 minutes until thickened. Remove from heat and stir in cream; stir until mixture stops bubbling. Stir in vanilla.

4. Arrange apple mixture over the crust. Top with the quartered caramels and drizzle with the caramel syrup. Bake for 25–30 minutes or until the apples are tender and the crust is light golden brown. Serve warm.

Nutrition Info: (Per Serving):Calories: 692; Total Fat: 24 g; Saturated Fat: 14 g; Cholesterol: 115 mg; Protein: 5 g; Sodium: 100 mg; Potassium: 214 mg; Fiber: 2 g; Carbohydrates: 118 g; Sugar: 60 g

Peanut Butter Brownies

Servings: 36 Bars

Ingredients:

- 13/4 cups unsalted peanut butter, divided
- 1/2 cup unsalted butter, softened
- 1 cup brown sugar
- 1 cup granulated sugar
- 3 large eggs, beaten
- 2 teaspoons vanilla
- 13/4 cups flour
- 1/2 teaspoon baking powder
- 1 cup chopped unsalted peanuts
- 1 (12-ounce) package semisweet chocolate chips

Directions:

1. Preheat oven to 325°F. Spray a 13" × 9" glass baking dish with nonstick baking spray containing flour and set aside.

2. In large bowl, combine 11/4 cups peanut butter and butter; mix until combined. Add brown sugar and granulated sugar and mix until combined.

3. Add eggs and beat until combined; do not overbeat. Mix in vanilla.

4. Stir in flour and baking powder and mix. Add the unsalted peanuts. Spoon into prepared pan and smooth top.

5. Bake for 30–35 minutes or until the bars are just set. Cool on wire rack for 30 minutes.

6. In small microwave-safe bowl, combine chocolate chips and remaining 1/2 cup peanut butter. Microwave on high power for 2 minutes, then remove and stir until chips are melted and mixture is smooth. Pour over brownies and spread to coat. Let stand until the glaze is set, then cut into bars.

Nutrition Info: (Per Serving):Calories: 237; Total Fat: 13 g; Saturated Fat: 3 g; Cholesterol: 24 mg; Protein: 5 g; Sodium: 15 mg; Potassium: 129 mg; Fiber: 1 g; Carbohydrates: 25 g; Sugar: 17 g

Butterscotch Pudding

Servings: 4

Ingredients:

- 2 tablespoons butter
- 2 tablespoons flour
- 1 tablespoon cornstarch
- 1 cup whole milk
- 1/3 cup light brown sugar
- 1/3 cup dark brown sugar
- 2 egg yolks
- 3/4 cup light cream
- 11/2 teaspoons vanilla

Directions:

1. In heavy saucepan, melt butter over medium heat. Add flour and cornstarch and cook for 1 minute until mixture bubbles, stirring constantly with a wire whisk.

2. Add milk and stir until smooth, making sure the whisk gets into the corners of the pan. Then add sugars, egg yolks, and light cream and, stirring constantly with a wire whisk, cook until mixture comes to a boil. Cook for another 2 minutes until thickened.

3. Remove from heat and add vanilla; whisk until smooth.

4. Cool, stirring occasionally, for about 40 minutes, then pour into serving dishes. Cover and chill for 1–2 hours before serving.

Nutrition Info: (Per Serving):Calories: 410; Total Fat: 23 g; Saturated Fat: 14 g; Cholesterol: 176 mg; Protein: 4 g; Sodium: 55 mg; Potassium: 196 mg; Fiber: 0 g; Carbohydrates: 45 g; Sugar: 38 g

Apple Cake

Servings: 24

Ingredients:

- 1 cup (235 ml) vegetable oil
- 2 cups (400 g) sugar
- 3 eggs
- 2 ½ cups (275 g) all-purpose flour
- 2 teaspoons (9 g) sodium-free baking powder
- 1 teaspoon sodium-free baking soda
- ½ teaspoon ground cinnamon
- ½ teaspoon ground nutmeg
- 1 teaspoon vanilla extract
- 3 cups (450 g) apples, peeled and chopped

Directions:

1. Mix oil and sugar together; add eggs. Sift together flour, baking powder, baking soda, cinnamon, and nutmeg; add to sugar mixture. Stir in vanilla and fold in apples. Pour into a 9 × 13-inch (23 × 33-cm) pan. Bake at 350°F (180°C, gas mark 4) until knife inserted in

center comes out clean, 1 to 1 ½ hours. Dust top with powdered sugar if desired.

Nutrition Info: (Per Serving): 19 g water; 211 calories (42% from fat, 4% from protein, 54% from carb); 2 g protein; 10 g total fat; 1 g saturated fat; 2 g monounsaturated fat; 5 g polyunsaturated fat; 29 g carb; 1 g fiber; 18 g sugar; 25 mg calcium; 1 mg iron; 11 mg sodium; 79 mg potassium; 41 IU vitamin A; 1 mg vitamin C; 31 mg cholesterol

Brownies

Servings: 24

Ingredients:

- ¾ cup (165 g) unsalted butter, melted
- 1 ½ cups (300 g) sugar
- 1 ½ teaspoons vanilla extract
- 3 eggs
- ½ cup (55 g) cocoa
- ¾ cup (83 g) all-purpose flour
- ½ teaspoon sodium-free baking powder
- 1 cup (175 g) chocolate chips

Directions:

1. Beat butter, sugar, vanilla, and eggs In a large bowl. Mix in cocoa, flour, and baking powder. Stir to Combine. Stir in chocolate chips. Pour into a greased 9 × 13-inch (23 × 33-cm) pan. Bake at 350°F (180°C, gas mark 4) for 20 to 22 minutes.

Nutrition Info: (Per Serving): 8 g water; 167 calories (46% from fat, 5% from protein, 49% from carb); 2 g protein; 9 g total fat; 5 g saturated fat; 3 g monounsaturated fat; 0 g polyunsaturated fat; 21 g carb; 1 g fiber; 16 g sugar; 26 mg calcium; 1 mg iron;

17 mg sodium; 80 mg potassium; 225 IU vitamin A; 0 mg vitamin C; 48 mg cholesterol

Angel Food Cake

Servings: 12

Ingredients:

- 11 egg whites, at room temperature
- 1 teaspoon cream of tartar
- 1/2 teaspoon lemon juice
- 11/4 cups granulated sugar
- 1/2 cup powdered sugar
- 1 cup cake flour
- 11/2 teaspoons vanilla

Directions:

1. Preheat oven to 325°F. Place the oven rack in the lowest position in the oven.
2. In large bowl, combine egg whites, cream of tartar, and lemon juice. Beat until soft peaks form.
3. Gradually beat in granulated sugar, about a tablespoon at a time, until the meringue is stiff and glossy. Beat in powdered sugar until combined.
4. Fold in half of the cake flour until combined, then fold in remaining flour. Stir in vanilla.

5. Spoon batter into an ungreased 10" angel food tube pan. Rap the pan on the counter gently once to remove any large air bubbles.

6. Bake for 40–50 minutes or until the cake is light golden brown and set. Immediately invert pan onto a bottle. It must cool upside down so the delicate structure doesn't collapse while cooling.

7. To remove from pan, run a sharp knife around the outside and around the center tube. Gently push cake out of pan. Turn onto serving plate.

Nutrition Info: (Per Serving):Calories: 145; Total Fat: 0 g; Saturated Fat: 0 g; Cholesterol: 0 mg; Protein: 1 g; Sodium: 5 mg; Potassium: 59 mg; Fiber: 0 g; Carbohydrates: 35 g; Sugar: 25 g

Chocolate Crackles

Servings: 40

Ingredients:

- 2 eggs
- 1 cup (200 g) sugar
- 1 teaspoon vanilla extract
- 3 ounces (85 g) unsweetened chocolate, grated
- 2 cups (200 g) unsalted pecans, finely chopped
- ¼ cup (30 g) dry low sodium bread crumbs
- 2 tablespoons (16 g) all-purpose flour
- ¾ teaspoon ground cinnamon
- ¼ cup (25 g) confectioners' sugar

Directions:

1. Beat eggs with sugar and vanilla to blend well. Mix in remaining ingredients except confectioners' sugar. If dough is soft, chill until it is easy to handle. Shape dough into 1-inch (2.5-cm) balls. Roll balls in confectioners' sugar and place 1 inch (2.5 cm) apart on greased baking sheet. Bake at 325°F (170°C, gas mark 3) for 12 to 15 minutes. They will be

soft and crackled on top. Cool on racks. Store in tightly covered container.

Nutrition Info: (Per Serving): 2 g water; 81 calories (58% from fat, 6% from protein, 37% from carb); 1 g protein; 6 g total fat; 1 g saturated fat; 3 g monounsaturated fat; 1 g polyunsaturated fat; 8 g carb; 1 g fiber; 6 g sugar; 9 mg calcium; 1 mg iron; 5 mg sodium; 45 mg potassium; 20 IU vitamin A; 0 mg vitamin C; 12 mg cholesterol

Cranberry Upside-down Cake

Servings: 12

Ingredients:

- 2 cups (220 g) cranberries
- 1 ¾ cups (350 g) sugar, divided
- ½ cup (120 ml) water
- 1 cup (110 g) all-purpose flour
- 1 ½ teaspoons sodium-free baking powder
- ½ cup (125 g) applesauce
- 1 egg
- ¼ cup (60 ml) skim milk
- ¼ cup (60 ml) orange juice
- 1 teaspoon orange peel, grated
- ½ teaspoon vanilla extract

Directions:

1. Spray bottom and sides of 9-inch (23-cm) round baking pan with nonstick vegetable oil spray. Combine cranberries, 1 cup (200 g) of the sugar, and the water In a large saucepan. Bring to a boil. Reduce heat and simmer until slightly thickened to syrupy consistency, about 10 minutes. Pour into prepared pan. Cool to room temperature.

2.   Sift together flour, remaining ¾ cup (150 g) sugar, and baking powder In a large bowl. In another bowl stir applesauce, egg, milk, orange juice, orange peel, and vanilla until blended. Add to dry ingredients and stir just until blended. Pour over cranberry mixture. Bake at 375°F (190°C, gas mark 5) for 25 to 30 minutes or until wooden pick inserted in center comes out clean. Let cake cool in pan about 5 minutes. Loosen cake around edges of pan. Place inverted serving platter over cake and turn both upside down. Shake gently, then remove pan. Serve warm.

Nutrition Info: (Per Serving): 37 g water; 255 calories (3% from fat, 4% from protein, 93% from carb); 3 g protein; 1 g total fat; 0 g saturated fat; 0 g monounsaturated fat; 0 g polyunsaturated fat; 62 g carb; 1 g fiber; 46 g sugar; 54 mg calcium; 1 mg iron; 17 mg sodium; 314 mg potassium; 40 IU vitamin A; 3 mg vitamin C; 21 mg cholesterol

Strawberry Basil Pie

Servings: 8

Ingredients:

- 1 recipe Cookie Pie Crust , baked and cooled
- 3 cups strawberry sorbet, slightly softened
- 1 tablespoon lemon juice
- 2 tablespoons chopped fresh basil leaves
- 2 cups sliced fresh strawberries

Directions:

1. Prepare cookie pie crust and let cool.
2. In large bowl, combine strawberry sorbet, lemon juice, and basil and mix until combined. Stir in fresh strawberries.
3. Pile into the pie crust and freeze until firm, about 4–6 hours. Let stand at room temperature for 15–20 minutes before serving for easier slicing.

Nutrition Info: (Per Serving):Calories: 275; Total Fat: 9 g; Saturated Fat: 5 g; Cholesterol: 46 mg; Protein: 3 g; Sodium: 29 mg; Potassium: 155 mg; Fiber: 2 g; Carbohydrates: 44 g; Sugar: 24 g

V6

Servings: 4

Ingredients:

- 2 cups (360 g) tomatoes
- ½ cup (70 g) cucumber
- ¼ cup (30 g) green bell peppers
- ¼ cup (25 g) celery
- ½ cup (130 g) carrot
- ¼ cup (15 g) parsley, fresh

Directions:

1. Cut all ingredients so that they easily fit into the juice extractor. Process all ingredients into juice extractor in the order given. Stir and enjoy.

Nutrition Info: (Per Serving): 112 g water; 25 calories (8% from fat, 15% from protein, 77% from carb); 1 g protein; 0 g total fat; 0 g saturated fat; 0 g monounsaturated fat; 0 g polyunsaturated fat; 6 g carb; 2 g fiber; 3 g sugar; 23 mg calcium; 1 mg iron; 23 mg sodium; 295 mg potassium; 2927 IU vitamin A; 20 mg vitamin C; 0 mg cholesterol

Blackberry Cobbler

Servings: 8

Ingredients:

- 2 tablespoons (16 g) cornstarch
- ¼ cup (60 ml) cold water
- 1 ½ cups (300 g) sugar, divided
- 1 tablespoon (15 ml) lemon juice
- 4 cups (580 g) blackberries
- 1 cup (110 g) all-purpose flour
- 1 teaspoon sodium-free baking powder
- 6 tablespoons (85 g) unsalted butter
- ¼ cup (60 ml) boiling water

Directions:

1. In a saucepan, stir together the cornstarch and cold water until cornstarch is completely dissolved. Add 1 cup (200 g) of the sugar, lemon juice, and blackberries; Combine gently. In a bowl, Combine the flour, remaining ½ cup (100 g) sugar, and baking powder. Blend in the butter until the mixture resembles coarse meal. Add the boiling water and stir the mixture until it just forms a dough. Bring the blackberry mixture to a boil,

stirring. Transfer to a 1 ½-quart (1 ½-L) baking dish. Drop spoonfuls of the dough carefully onto the mixture, and bake the cobbler on a baking sheet in the middle of a preheated 400°F (200°C, gas mark 6) oven for 20 to 25 minutes, or until the topping is golden.

Nutrition Info: (Per Serving): 84 g water; 319 calories (25% from fat, 3% from protein, 72% from carb); 3 g protein; 9 g total fat; 6 g saturated fat; 2 g monounsaturated fat; 1 g polyunsaturated fat; 59 g carb; 4 g fiber; 41 g sugar; 54 mg calcium; 1 mg iron; 3 mg sodium; 202 mg potassium; 420 IU vitamin A; 16 mg vitamin C; 23 mg cholesterol

Cookie Pie Crust

Servings: 8

Ingredients:

- 1/3 cup unsalted butter
- 1/4 cup granulated sugar
- 2 tablespoons brown sugar
- 1 egg yolk
- 1 teaspoon vanilla
- 1/2 teaspoon grated lemon zest
- 11/4 cups flour

Directions:

1. Preheat oven to 350°F. In medium bowl, combine butter with granulated sugar and brown sugar and mix well. Beat in egg yolk, vanilla, and lemon zest.
2. Add flour and mix until a dough forms.
3. Press into the bottom and up the sides of 9" pie pan. Flute edge if desired. Prick bottom of crust with fork.
4. Bake for 12–15 minutes or until the pie crust is light golden brown. Let cool completely and fill as desired.

Nutrition Info: (Per Serving):Calories: 180; Total Fat: 8 g; Saturated Fat: 5 g; Cholesterol: 46 mg; Protein: 2 g; Sodium: 3 mg; Potassium: 30 mg; Fiber: 0 g; Carbohydrates: 23 g; Sugar: 8 g

Strawberry Iced Tea Fizz

Servings: 12

Ingredients:

- 1 quart (1 L) strawberries, sliced
- ½ cup (100 g) sugar
- 5 cups (1175 ml) water, boiling
- 1 tea bag
- 12 ounces (340 g) frozen lemonade concentrate, thawed
- 1 quart (1 L) seltzer water

Directions:

1. In large bowl, Combine strawberries and sugar; set aside. In another bowl, pour water over tea bag; steep 5 minutes. Discard tea bag; cool tea to room temperature. Stir tea into strawberry mixture along with lemonade concentrate; chill. To serve, stir in sparkling water and ladle over ice cubes in tall glasses. Serve with spoons.

Nutrition Info: (Per Serving): 259 g water; 110 calories (1% from fat, 1% from protein, 98% from carb); 0 g protein; 0 g total fat; 0 g saturated fat; 0 g monounsaturated fat; 0 g polyunsaturated fat; 28 g carb; 2 g fiber; 25 g sugar; 27 mg calcium; 1 mg iron; 5 mg sodium; 128 mg potassium; 35 IU vitamin A; 35 mg vitamin C; 0 mg cholesterol

Strawberry Smoothie

Servings: 2

Ingredients:

- 1 ¼ cups (152 g) strawberries
- 1 ½ cups (295 ml) skim milk
- 1 tablespoon (13 g) sugar
- 1 teaspoon lemon juice

Directions:

1. Put all ingredients in a blender and process until smooth.

Nutrition Info: (Per Serving): 254 g water; 131 calories (5% from fat, 24% from protein, 71% from carb); 8 g protein; 1 g total fat; 0 g saturated fat; 0 g monounsaturated fat; 0 g polyunsaturated fat; 24 g carb; 2 g fiber; 11 g sugar; 279 mg calcium; 1 mg iron; 110 mg sodium; 484 mg potassium; 386 IU vitamin A; 59 mg vitamin C; 4 mg cholesterol

Triple Berry Pavlova

Servings: 6

Ingredients:

- 5 egg whites
- 1/2 teaspoon lemon juice
- 1 cup sugar
- 2 teaspoons cornstarch
- 1 teaspoon apple cider vinegar
- 1 1/2 teaspoons vanilla, divided
- 1/2 cup heavy whipping cream
- 3 tablespoons powdered sugar
- 1/2 cup Lemon Curd
- 1 cup raspberries
- 1 cup blueberries
- 1 cup blackberries
- 2 tablespoons orange juice

Directions:

1. Preheat oven to 300°F.
2. In large bowl, place egg whites and lemon juice; beat until soft peaks form. Gradually add sugar, about a tablespoon at a time, beating until the meringue holds a stiff peak.

3. Stir in cornstarch, vinegar, and 1 teaspoon vanilla.

4. Place parchment paper on a baking sheet. Spoon the meringue onto the sheet, creating a 9" circle; smooth the top. Bake for 50–60 minutes or until the meringue is crisp on the outside. Cool on the paper on a wire rack.

5. When ready to eat, peel the paper off the meringue and turn it over onto a serving plate so the top is on the bottom.

6. In medium bowl, beat whipping cream with powdered sugar and remaining 1/2 teaspoon vanilla until soft peaks form. Fold in lemon curd. Pile this mixture on the meringue.

7. Top with berries and drizzle with orange juice. Refrigerate for an hour or two, or serve immediately.

Nutrition Info: (Per Serving):Calories: 317; Total Fat: 10 g; Saturated Fat: 6 g; Cholesterol: 59 mg; Protein: 5 g; Sodium: 63 mg; Potassium: 178 mg; Fiber: 3 g; Carbohydrates: 53 g; Sugar: 47 g

Pie Crust

Servings: 8

Ingredients:

- ⅓ cup (80 ml) vegetable oil
- 1 ⅓ cups (147 g) all-purpose flour
- 2 tablespoons (28 ml) water, cold

Directions:

1. Add oil to flour and mix well with fork. Sprinkle water over and mix well. With hands, press into ball and flatten. Roll between two pieces of waxed paper. Remove top waxed paper, invert over pan, and remove other paper. Press into place. For pies that do not require a baked filling, bake at 400°F (200°C, gas mark 6) until lightly browned, 12 to 15 minutes.

Nutrition Info: (Per Serving): 6 g water; 156 calories (54% from fat, 6% from protein, 41% from carb); 2 g protein; 9 g total fat; 1 g saturated fat; 2 g monounsaturated fat; 5 g polyunsaturated fat; 16 g carb; 1 g fiber; 0 g sugar; 3 mg calcium; 1 mg iron; 0 mg sodium; 22 mg potassium; 0 IU vitamin A; 0 mg vitamin C; 0 mg cholesterol

Tomato Juice

Servings: 4

Ingredients:

- 6 ounces (170 g) no-salt-added tomato paste
- 1 ½ cups (355 ml) water
- 1 tablespoon (15 ml) hot pepper sauce

Directions:

1. Blend and chill.

Nutrition Info: (Per Serving): 123 g water; 35 calories (5% from fat, 18% from protein, 77% from carb); 2 g protein; 0 g total fat; 0 g saturated fat; 0 g monounsaturated fat; 0 g polyunsaturated fat; 8 g carb; 2 g fiber; 4 g sugar; 18 mg calcium; 1 mg iron; 66 mg sodium; 436 mg potassium; 706 IU vitamin A; 9 mg vitamin C; 1 mg cholesterol

Strawberry Rhubarb Raspberry Crisp

Servings: 8

Ingredients:

- 2 cups sliced fresh rhubarb
- 2 cups sliced strawberries
- 2 cups raspberries
- 3/4 cup sugar
- 1 cup plus 2 tablespoons flour, divided
- 2 tablespoons lemon juice
- 1/2 teaspoon grated lemon zest
- 11/2 cups rolled oats
- 1 cup brown sugar
- 1/2 cup chopped pecans
- 3/4 cup unsalted butter, melted
- 1/2 teaspoon cinnamon

Directions:

1. Preheat oven to 375°F. Spray a 9" × 13" glass baking dish with nonstick cooking spray containing flour and set aside.

2. Combine rhubarb, strawberries, and raspberries in the baking dish. Sprinkle with sugar, 2 tablespoons flour, lemon juice, and zest and toss gently to coat.

3. In medium bowl, combine remaining 1 cup flour, rolled oats, brown sugar, and pecans, and mix well. Add melted butter and cinnamon and mix until crumbly. Spoon on top of the fruit.

4. Bake for 40–50 minutes or until fruit mixture is bubbly and tender and the streusel topping is golden brown. Let cool 1 hour, then serve.

Nutrition Info: (Per Serving):Calories: 534; Total Fat: 23 g; Saturated Fat: 11 g; Cholesterol: 45 mg; Protein: 5 g; Sodium: 12 mg; Potassium: 349 mg; Fiber: 6 g; Carbohydrates: 79 g; Sugar: 50 g

Snickerdoodles

Servings: 72

Ingredients:

- 1 cup (225 g) unsalted butter
- 1 ½ cups (300 g) sugar
- 2 eggs
- 1 teaspoon vanilla extract
- 2 ⅔ cups (293 g) all-purpose flour
- 2 teaspoons cream of tartar
- 2 teaspoons (9 g) sodium-free baking soda
- 2 tablespoons (26 g) sugar
- 1 teaspoon ground cinnamon

Directions:

1. Cream butter until light. Add 1 ½ cups (300 g) sugar and beat until fluffy. Beat in eggs and vanilla. Stir together flour, cream of tartar, and baking soda. Add to beaten mixture. Stir together 2 tablespoons (26 g) sugar and cinnamon. Shape dough into 1-inch (2.5-cm) balls. Roll in cinnamon-sugar mixture. Place 2 inches (5 cm) apart on ungreased baking

sheet. Bake at 400°F (200°C, gas mark 6) for 8 to 10 minutes. Remove and cool on racks.

Nutrition Info: (Per Serving): 2 g water; 60 calories (41% from fat, 5% from protein, 54% from carb); 1 g protein; 3 g total fat; 2 g saturated fat; 1 g monounsaturated fat; 0 g polyunsaturated fat; 8 g carb; 0 g fiber; 5 g sugar; 3 mg calcium; 0 mg iron; 3 mg sodium; 22 mg potassium; 87 IU vitamin A; 0 mg vitamin C; 14 mg cholesterol

Baked Apples

Servings: 4

Ingredients:

- 2 large apples, cored and cut in half
- 2 teaspoons lemon juice
- 4 teaspoons brown sugar
- 4 teaspoons rolled oats
- Nonstick cooking spray
- 1/8 cup water

Directions:

1. Preheat oven to 375°F. Treat an ovenproof dish with nonstick cooking spray.

2. Place the apples cut-side up in the prepared dish. Brush 1 teaspoon of the lemon juice over each apple half.

3. In a small bowl, mix together the brown sugar and rolled oats; evenly divide over the apples. Mist the top of the apples with the cooking spray.

4. Add the water to the bottom of the baking dish. Bake for 35 minutes or until the apples are fork tender. Serve hot or cold.

Nutrition Info: (Per Serving):Calories: 70; Total Fat: 0 g; Saturated Fat: 0 g; Cholesterol: 0 mg; Protein: 0 g; Sodium: 0 mg; Potassium: 110 mg; Fiber: 1 g; Carbohydrates: 18 g; Sugar: 14 g

Fruit Sauce

Servings: 4

Ingredients:

- 1 teaspoon ground cinnamon
- 4 teaspoons vanilla sugar
- 11/2 teaspoons rosewater
- 11/2 teaspoons orange flower water
- 4 teaspoons unsalted butter

Directions:

1. In a small microwave-safe bowl, combine the cinnamon, sugar, and flower waters; microwave on high for 30 seconds.
2. Stir until the sugar is dissolved, then whisk in the butter. Serve immediately.

Nutrition Info: (Per Serving):Calories: 51; Total Fat: 3 g; Saturated Fat: 2 g; Cholesterol: 10 mg; Protein: 0 g; Sodium: 0 mg; Potassium: 4 mg; Fiber: 0 g; Carbohydrates: 4 g; Sugar: 4 g

Venison And Veggie Stovetop Casserole

Servings: 4

Ingredients:

- 1 teaspoon olive oil
- 1 teaspoon butter
- 1 small sweet onion, chopped
- 1/2 cup no-salt-added tomato purée
- 2 cloves garlic, minced
- 1/4 teaspoon low-sodium beef base
- 3/4 cup dry red wine
- 2 tablespoons red currant jelly
- 1/2 cup water
- 1/8 cup lemon juice
- 1 tablespoon cornstarch
- Optional: 1/4 teaspoon granulated sugar
- 1/4 teaspoon dried parsley
- 1/8 teaspoon salt-free chili powder
- 1/8 teaspoon mustard powder
- 1/8 teaspoon freshly ground black pepper
- Pinch dried thyme
- Pinch dried basil

- 1 (16-ounce) package frozen hash brown potatoes, thawed
- 1 (10-ounce) frozen vegetable blend, thawed
- 1 pound Slow-Cooked Venison, cubed
- Optional: Fresh parsley sprigs

Directions:

1. Heat the olive oil and butter in a large, deep nonstick sauté pan. Add the onion and sauté until transparent; stir in the tomato purée and sauté for 2 minutes. Add the garlic and sauté for 1 minute. Add the beef base; stir to dissolve and mix it with the other ingredients.

2. In a mixing cup, whisk together the wine, jelly, water, lemon juice, and cornstarch. Add to the pan and bring to a boil.

3. Add the sugar, if using, parsley, chili powder, mustard powder, pepper, thyme, basil, and hash browns; stir to coat. Reduce heat, cover, and simmer for 30 minutes.

4. Add the thawed vegetables and meat; simmer for 5–10 minutes longer until heated through. Serve immediately, garnished with fresh parsley, if desired.

Nutrition Info: (Per Serving):Calories: 364; Total Fat: 6 g; Saturated Fat: 1 g; Cholesterol: 90 mg; Protein: 27 g; Sodium: 133 mg; Potassium: 985 mg; Fiber: 5 g; Carbohydrates: 41 g; Sugar: 5 g

Pork Tenderloin Bruschetta

Servings: 4

Ingredients:

- 1 pound pork tenderloin
- 1 tablespoon olive oil
- 1 teaspoon dried basil leaves
- 1/4 teaspoon pepper
- 2 beefsteak tomatoes, seeded and chopped
- 1 shallot, minced
- 1 clove garlic, minced
- 1/3 cup sliced fresh basil leaves
- 2 tablespoons lemon juice
- 2 tablespoons extra-virgin olive oil

Directions:

1. Slice the tenderloin into 4 pieces, slicing across the tenderloin but at an angle. Press on the pieces until they are about 1" thick. Brush with olive oil and sprinkle with dried basil and pepper.
2. In medium bowl, combine tomatoes, shallot, garlic, basil, lemon juice, and extra-virgin olive oil; mix well and refrigerate.

3. Prepare and preheat grill. Grill the tenderloin slices 6" from medium coals for 4–6 minutes per side, turning once, until a meat thermometer registers at least 145°F. Top each piece with some of the cold tomato mixture and serve immediately.

Nutrition Info: (Per Serving):Calories: 222; Total Fat: 12 g; Saturated Fat: 2 g; Cholesterol: 73 mg; Protein: 24 g; Sodium: 62 mg; Potassium: 549 mg; Fiber: 0 g; Carbohydrates: 2 g; Sugar: 1 g